INTERMITTENT FASTING

10 MOST COMMON MISTAKES YOU SHOULD KNOW ABOUT

Jennifer J Collins

I want to dedicate this book to all those who have supported us during all this year, especially to my dear and beloved family.

Dedicate it to all my friend and to all of you who acquired this book,

I hope that all the information in this work will be of great help to all of you, that all your goals and objectives will be achieved and that you will look better every day, with the quality of life that you deserve.

Do not forget that you are a unique person and do not care what people tell you,
you have a lot of courage.

CONTENIDO

Página del título

Dedicatoria

Introducción

grattitude 1

THE INTERMITTENT FASTING 3

What is intermittent fasting? 4

Ketogenic Diet 10

Dieting for the right reasons 14

1º You don't drink enough water 17

2º You are going at a fast pace 19

3º You don't take care of the electrolytes 21

4º You don't eat enough 22

5º You maintain a high carbohydrate diet 24

6º Tomas excess snacks 26

7º You take collagen in your coffee Keto 28

8º You are not flexible with your feeding window 30

9º You drink alcohol outside your food window 32

10º You don't sleep enough 34

INTRODUCCIÓN

◆ ◆ ◆

THE INTERMITTENT FASTING

We love intermittent fasting here I will show you 10 mistakes that people often make and that you should know The intermittent fasting for an easy way together with the Keto diet to lose weight without difficulties, but there are several mistakes you can make when doing the intermittent fasting.

"Intermittent fasting consists of establishing more specific time intervals for meals and between 12 and 16 hours of fasting per day", intermittent or sporadic fasting are more common daily (at least 12 hours of fasting, the best known pattern being "16/8"), there are others, such as weekly (usually one or two days a week of fasting, followed or not). Within this second option, the most popular is the so-called "5:2 diet", which advocates eating normally five days a week and a severe reduction in intake (over 75%) the next two. Fasting on a monthly basis (fasting a couple of days in a row each month) is practised to a lesser extent.

GRATTITUDE

◆ ◆ ◆

Of all the recipes for achieving abundance and prosperity in our lives, the best we can practice is gratitude.

Because feeling a sincere gratitude for what you have automatically and if effort, rather be to your life,

That's why it's so important for you to start now to value and recognize all the blessings you've already received.

Even if you cannot see it physically yet, that is why I am going to express here my gratitude that I have long expressed every morning when I got up and that has allowed me to be more grateful and to stay in the frequency of daily abundance and prosperity.

Being grateful brings me benefit when I close my eyes and expressed with sincerity, really feeling the gratitude in your heart.

Knowing that the creator God of the universe is conspiring to give you what you desire.

Dear God thank you for this day, I thank you for allowing me to experience this magical moment in my life.

Thank you for my family for my friends and my loved ones. Thank you for my health and well-being. For all the functions of my body that are performed to perfection.

Thank you for my house and everything in it. Thank you for all my possessions and for my home aspect of my life.

Thanks,

Because I appreciate all that I am today. For the morning sun, for the birds singing and the flowers in the morning.

Thank you for all the beauty that surrounds me at this time. Thank you for the prosperity I receive and will receive multiplied.

Thanks for every smile I will see and receive today. For all the blessings I will enjoy today.

For the opportunities that are unfolding before me. I choose to radiate gratitude to everyone and do everything I contacted today.

My heart is filled with recognition and thanksgiving for all you have given me and for the opportunity to help many people achieve happiness and feel better every day.

My God, thank you for opening my heart. Thank you for the wonderful gift again.

My God, thank you for the wonderful gift of my life.

Jennifer J Collins

THE INTERMITTENT FASTING

◆ ◆ ◆

We love intermittent fasting here I will show you 10 mistakes that people often make and that you should know.

The intermittent fasting for an easy way together with the Keto diet to lose weight without difficulties, but there are several mistakes you can make when doing the intermittent fasting.

"Intermittent fasting consists of establishing more specific time intervals for meals and between 12 and 16 hours of fasting per day", intermittent or sporadic fasting are more common daily (at least 12 hours of fasting, the best known pattern being "16/8"), there are others, such as weekly (usually one or two days a week of fasting, followed or not). Within this second option, the most popular is the so-called "5:2 diet", which advocates eating normally five days a week and a severe reduction in intake (over 75%) the next two. Fasting on a monthly basis (fasting a couple of days in a row each month) is practiced to a lesser extent.

WHAT IS INTERMITTENT FASTING?

Why does it help you lose weight?

How about the idea of fasting without putting too much effort into it? Everything you need to know about intermittent fasting.

Intermitten t Fasting, or IFA, is the most popular weight loss program today, and many celebrities, such as Hugh Jackman, Chris Hemsworth, and even Benedict Cumberbatch, have jumped on the Intermittent Fasting bandwagon.

And Bing's doctor in Raw, a primary care physician, said he lost 100 pounds (ca. 45 kg) in just 18 months thanks to Intermittent Fasting.

Before he tried the technique he weighed 300 pounds (0.14 t), so it seems that intermittent fasting is a real miracle.

What is the secret behind it that makes it so effective? Let's unravel the truth of this weight loss madness with a question that lingers in our minds.

Is it possible that the human body can endure long hours without food daily? Let's investigate a little first who created intermittent fasting.

In general, it is an ancient practice but it has nothing to do with your dream of achieving a perfect body to go to the beach in fact, humans have done things like that all their lives.

Important Greek personalities such as Pythagoras, Socrates and Plato helped to purify their spirit and mind.

Some major religions practice fasting to strengthen their faith. Mahatma Gandhi, fasting 17 times during his campaigns for India's independence, not only lost a few pounds but also overthrew the British government.

But when fasting gained recognition as a means of losing weight was popularized by the American writer Upton Sinclair, in the 20th century he practiced juice cleanliness and fasting simultaneously.

In August 2012 fasting gained recognition from the health and fitness community thanks to the influence of doctor and journalist Michael Moss Lee, he published a book on the subject in January 2013 entitled the fasting diet.

Before we continue we need to clear up misconceptions about this technique.

Firstly, intermittent fasting is often considered to be a type of diet, with intermittent fasting you do not control what you eat but take care when you do.

It is not a diet plan but a feeding pattern, we will explain this later in detail, for now, let's move on to the next myth of intermittent fasting.

The second misconception about this practice is that you must starve yourself, if we look in the dictionary for the meaning of hungry we'll read; "Intense and prolonged food shortage" on the other hand fasting means; "Total or partial deprivation of food for a while"

With him there you still have to eat and drink but it must be in a limited time.

That's why intermittent fasting is also considered a restricted feeding.

In time the third and final mistake that prevents health enthusiasts from trying this controversial weight loss program is the safety and well-being problems associated with intermittent fasting.

Let's get to the bottom of this by discussing how this technique works.

We mentioned earlier that intermittent fasting is a pattern of eating with fasting your entire day or week divided into two parts.

The feeding period and the fasting period, during the feeding period you can eat a regular meal, so if you don't need to starve.

During the fasting period you are not allowed to eat any food. No! Not a single bite can touch your lips.

But there is an exception to this rule during the fasting period you can drink but only water, tea or coffee without sugar or cream, please. In some cases you can eat hundreds of calories or a combo of fruits and vegetables while you are in fasting mode.

How can you divide your day or week into a meal period and a fasting period?

Can it be 2 hours of fasting and 22 hours of eating? It doesn't work like that, that's not an intermittent fast. That's compulsive eating.

The eating patterns you can follow are the 16-8 pattern, also known as "leangains" which was invented by fitness expert Martin Beckham "leangains" is an ideal fasting schedule for beginners, no kidding.

This method involves fasting for 14-16 hours per day, the remaining 6-8 hours are for the feeding period. The 5:2 pattern "the fasting diet" method created by British physician and journalist Michael Mosley if the same subject who revived the popularity of intermittent fasting.

This is lighter than the "leangains" protocol because you can eat 500 to 600 calories or high-calorie foods during the 2 days of fasting. And then you can eat naturally for 5 days. "Eat Stop

Eat was created by fitness expert Brad Bailey with this intermittent fasting eating pattern, you have to fast for 24 hours.

Once or twice a week for example you can start your fast on Monday at 12 pm and it will end on Tuesday the next day at 12 pm.

Alternating day fasting as the name suggests is when you fast every day and a half is a fasting period in a fasting period you can eat 500 to 600 calories or nothing at all.

The Warrior Diet It was popularized by fitness expert Ori Hofmekler this method requires fasting all day.

You can still eat small portions of fruits and vegetables. The feeding period is from 6 pm to 10 pm and you can eat a large meal.

The main concern about intermittent fasting is the large amount of time required for the fasting period. We are scheduled to eat breakfast, lunch, dinner, and a couple of snacks throughout the day.

How would your body feel if you skipped any of these meals? You may experience hunger, weakness, dizziness, or vomiting. You may also have sudden mood swings.

How to go from frustration to irritation are normal bodily reactions during the first few weeks or months of fasting.

That's because the body is still adjusting to the new regimen. What can fasting really accomplish? Over time your body will eventually overcome the side effects, under normal circumstances your body gets energy from the food you eat. This is stored in your liver and muscles.

What about when you are fasting? Your body gets fuel from its last reserve.

The stored fats are burned to become energy the longer you fast, the more fat will be burned in the process.

What are the other health benefits of this technique besides helping your body get rid of unwanted pounds?

Good,

> Can prevent type 2 diabetes
> Promote insulin resistance
> Good for the heart, may prevent cancer
> Improves brain function
> It promotes longevity and simplifies your lifestyle.

Because you don't have to plan to cook or pack 3-6 meals a day you can save money and time when shopping and preparing food. Hey! That means fewer dishes to wash up too.

Although intermittent fasting looks promising, this weight loss solution is not for everyone. If you really want to try the technique, we suggest that you consult your doctor first.

Especially in these cases; Diabetes low blood pressure Pregnancy or attempted pregnancy History of eating disorders.

In addition, children and adolescents are advised not to try fasting, because at this stage of their development they need more energy than adults. You must also remember that you cannot lose weight through intermittent fasting alone.

Because you are always fasting, your body needs adequate nutrition from healthy foods such as dairy, lean protein, nuts and seeds, vegetables, whole grains, and whole and unprocessed foods. It's also safe to exercise while fasting, but we recommend exercising after your body has adjusted and you don't have any side effects such as hunger or weakness. It's hard to lose weight no matter what weight loss program you choose - sacrifices have to be made.

Saying goodbye to your favorite fatty foods or not eating at all once in a while. Keep in mind that you should check with your doctor before starting any activity - intermittent fasting may work for others but may not be right for you. It's not because you can't keep away from that bag and you're either not self-controlled enough. It may have something to do with your body's constitution - don't despair - there are other weight loss programs besides intermittent fasting that you can mix and match like the Keto diet.

KETOGENIC DIET

◆ ◆ ◆

It's very fashionable these days if you've heard of the ketogenic diet or "Keto", as it's known in English. It's become very popular over the last few years.

There are more and more publications about it, and the interest on the internet is very high.   But what exactly is the ketogenic diet?

What does ketogenic mean, to begin with? And how is it done? In this course you will learn everything you need to know about it.

First, let's get something straight. What does the word "ketogenic" mean?

Basically, it has to do with the fact that the body can function on two types of fuels.

One is the sugar in the carbohydrates in the food we eat, which is the main fuel used by most people today.

For example, when you eat bread, pasta, rice, potatoes, etc. The other fuel is fat.   The ketogenic diet is a very low carbohydrate diet.

So low in carbohydrates, the body has to switch to using fat as the main fuel.

For example, fat from natural foods such as eggs, meat, avocados, butter, olive oil, nuts, etc.

Even the brain can get energy from fats. When the body runs out of sugar, the liver converts the fat into energy molecules called ketones, which provide the brain with energy.

And the diet that allows this is called ketogenic, since it produces ketones.

This is where the name of this type of diet comes from. Obtaining energy mainly from fat, a state known as "ketosis", has many benefits.

For example, it turns you into a fat-burning machine. In this state you lose weight without going hungry because you burn fat all the time, even when you sleep. And because it gives you enormous amounts of energy.

As to why the ketogenic diet has become super popular in recent years: It's really nothing new.

Its foundations have been built up over a long period of time. It's a strict low ketogenic, gluten-free diet, and it's similar to the Paleolithic diet.

It also looks a lot like the old, well-known Atkins diet. The basic idea is basic, and is that it is based on natural foods, simply avoid foods; such as sugar, fast and processed foods, bread, pasta, rice, etc.

Instead, you eat meat, fish, eggs, vegetables and natural fats, such as butter.

What's different about the ketogenic diet? That it is an ultra-improved low ketogenic diet, from which you can be sure you will get maximum benefits.

We'll get to the details later.

But, as I was saying, the ketogenic diet is an ultra-improved version of an old idea.

Similar diets have been tried for decades, even centuries. These similar diets are becoming increasingly well known because they work.

This might have an evolutionary explanation, since our ancestors didn't eat refined foods, or sugar the way we do today; so our bodies may not be adapted to those foods. Modern science shows that it works.

On a ketogenic diet, most people can lose excess weight without going hungry, and multiple health problems, such as insulin resistance, diabetes, or obesity, among others, tend to improve.

Most importantly, the ketogenic diet is not just used as a temporary solution.

Many people enjoy it as a lasting lifestyle.

Not just for weight loss, but for long-term health and well-being and for staying in shape all year round.

Many people feel energetic, full of energy and lucidity, and have stable blood sugar levels.

Hunger disappears, cravings for sweet foods are reduced, so

there's no need to be eating frequently anymore.

Time is saved by being satisfied with fewer meals per day. You eat delicious food every time you are hungry, and you don't even have to count calories.

Most people feel so full on the ketogenic diet that they can eat every time they are hungry, and still eat less and reduce excess weight.

DIETING FOR THE RIGHT REASONS

◆ ◆ ◆

When it comes to dieting, too often we take those first steps toward the happiness of weight loss for what we later determine are all the wrong reasons.

Ultimately, however, if your reason works for you, there is no truly wrong reason to diet.

The trick is to find the reason that really works for you. I have seen all kinds of excellent motivators when it comes to dieting and taking it seriously.

One of the most common reasons is to lose weight. This is as good a reason as any.

Some want to go back to the size 5 jeans they wore in high school, while others just want to be able to look at themselves in the mirror one more time without feeling guilty.

For some this is simply a matter of vanity and for others it is finally the handling of what has become a lifelong problem.

If you find the inspiration you need to succeed with your diet this time instead of others, then that is the perfectly plausible and acceptable reason for you to diet, and apply the intermittent fast.

Other reasons for dieting include the desire to be more fit.

Some of us have a deep and abiding desire to live as long as possible, and we firmly believe that the best possible method of achieving this goal is to live the healthiest life possible.

This is another great reason to lose weight and get in shape. If it works for you, that is. The thing to remember is that each person is going to have to find their motivation deep within themselves.

Another great reason is to have the energy you need to keep up with your little ones.

This is one of the most heartbreaking side effects for most when it comes to obesity.

There is simply no energy left at the end of the day to enjoy doing things with your precious little ones who are young for such a short time.

You desperately want to be able to build those precious memories with them, but you don't have the energy to do it.

If that's not bad enough, you've probably noticed (if you're considered morbidly obese) that many of the simplest activities with your kids often bring you physical pain that is a direct result of their weight.

Revenge is a dish best served cold and another excellent motivator for some when it comes to dieting and taking off those pesky pounds.

Losing a large amount of weight takes time in many cases, so you should be able to maintain your motivation even when things go wrong along the way.

The road to a new body is not an easy one. This is for those who have serious emotional healing to do and the best revenge for old slights and injuries is to become more beautiful than ever before.

If this motivation is what it takes for you to take off the pounds, then this is the motivation you must hold on to.

Religion is another common motivation for losing weight. Some people believe that the body should be treated like a temple.

There is nothing wrong with this philosophy at all, although it takes some of us longer than others to find our way along that line of thought.

Religion and faith are powerful motivations, as they have been known to bring healing to those in need through the power of their faith or their prayers.

If your faith can give you the willpower and strength you need to achieve your dieting and weight loss goals, then certainly, lean on your faith and keep it close.

No matter what motivation you have for dieting and weight loss if you find that it no longer works, then you must quickly find another motivator.

Without the right motivation, it is highly unlikely that you will be able to meet your weight loss goals.

I want to be the person who helps you most to reach your goals and definitely change your life because I've been in your shoes and I understand you completely.

1º YOU DON'T DRINK ENOUGH WATER

◆ ◆ ◆

Practicing intermittent fasting means that your body must spend a considerable number of hours at least 16 hours without any type of food that provides hydration or helps to keep water in the body.

This can cause dehydration, uncontrollable hunger, dizziness, weakness and muscle cramps, not to mention thirst.

This feeling will also make you feel irritated, perhaps a little confused, and you may start to consider throwing in the towel.

But it is not necessary to go to the extremes of getting sick and giving up fasting when everything can be easily solved by increasing your water consumption during the fasting hours.

The recommended amount of water a person should drink daily is eight glasses, but if you don't have food to help keep all that water in your body, it's normal to need to drink even more water than usual, especially since you are urinating more.

One way to help the body maintain hydration is to add a pinch of sea salt to the water. This secret that followers of the ketogenic diet apply, allows the body to retain water longer which reduces the possibility of dehydration.

During the intermittent fasting few drinks are allowed, only water, black coffee or black tea can know, and you cannot spend the day drinking tea or coffee, as they are stimulating drinks cannot get you rest at night.

If you are one of those people who enjoy their Keto coffee before eating, just when you start to break the fast, then we tell you that even before breaking the fast you should also drink a glass of water, since water helps to reduce the space available in the stomach for food, which will allow you to consume fewer calories.

In addition, one of the advantages of increasing water intake during the hours of fasting, is that it gives you satiety, which gives you a wonderful joker to resist those sudden attacks of hungering fact, in most cases that feeling of uncontrollable hunger are due more to thirst than the need for food.

2º YOU ARE GOING AT A FAST PACE

◆ ◆ ◆

It is good that the fasting hours, in the more sustainable mode of intermittent fasting, are 16 hours, but what is not good is that you try to complete the 16 hours from the beginning.

This will make you feel that it is going to be an impossible race towards an unattainable goal.

To be able to resist the 16 hours of fasting, babies should start at the bottom from about 10 hours of fasting initially, preferably at night so that most of the year is not spent sleeping and is not so difficult to sustain.

This doesn't mean that fasting for long hours is counterproductive, but that an organism accustomed to a high-carbohydrate diet, and with often frequent and irregular meal times, will feel shocked when it begins to lack the usual foods.

Not receiving the usual amounts of food, and on traditional schedules, the feeling of hunger increases,

This is because ghrelin, the hormone that tells the brain when to eat, is automatically activated, and its level increases when you check that leptin, the hormone that tells the brain when it is associated is not yet activated.

That's why the hunger wave can come suddenly and last for a long time in the first days, until it forces you to eat or lowers its intensity.

Therefore, it is not advisable to fast for 16 hours from the beginning because this feeling of hunger will make you feel bad and irritated.

The best thing is to start gradually, fasting first for about 10 hours, the next day for 11, and then you can increase the hours until you reach 16.

If you see that it doesn't work, you can practice a 12:12 fast for a week, this gives your body the possibility to adapt calmly and thus be able to advance.

3º YOU DON'T TAKE CARE
OF THE ELECTROLYTES

◆ ◆ ◆

Electrolytes are the tiny micronutrients that allow the body to stay in balance, regulating body functions such as keeping water in the body, blood pH, muscle functions and more.

The main electrolytes in the body are; chlorine, sodium and potassium, followed by other essential ones such as calcium, magnesium and phosphorus.

As you can imagine, fasting also reduces the supply of these electrolytes to the body, which can make you feel tired, thirsty, dehydrated or even have muscle pain or cramps.

This is why it is important to always keep yourself hydrated during the hours of fasting, but it also provides the body with an extra dose of electrolytes, which you can achieve with a pinch of sea salt in the water, or by taking a magnesium supplement.

Also remember to keep a healthy diet in your food window, including lots of green leafy vegetables gives you a high intake of minerals.

4º YOU DON'T EAT ENOUGH

◆ ◆ ◆

During the feeding window, your calorie intake needs to be lower than what you usually consume, but this does not mean that you should eat exaggeratedly small amounts of food.

One of the keys to intermittent fasting is that the food you eat should be healthy, rich in vegetables, protein and fat, and also socially rewarding.

To do this, you must eat until you feel full at the two or three meals you can eat during the feeding window.

If you don't eat until you are satisfied, especially during the last hour of your meal, ghrelin plays a role in finding you, making you feel hungry in advance and turning your fasting hours into a living hell for you and those around you because you are likely to be in a bad mood.

When you open your feeding window it is important that the first foods you make are proteins, that will help you replenish glycogen and provide substrate and energy to your muscles.

You should also consume fats and vegetables, especially

green leafy ones, and only if you are not completely satisfied can you consume unrefined carbohydrates.

5º YOU MAINTAIN A HIGH CARBOHYDRATE DIET

When you keep a high carbohydrate intake in your feeding window, you are playing against yourself.

One of the purposes of intermittent fasting is to reduce blood glucose levels so that the body can actually use its resources to burn fat effectively.

But this does not happen if you maintain a high-carbohydrate diet. Remember that this type of food provides the body with glucose, which, when not burned, is converted into fat and accumulates in the adipose tissue.

In addition, carbohydrates, especially refined ones, give you a momentary feeling of satiety, but then leave you with an even greater sense of hunger, which will make it very difficult to resist the hours of fasting.

This is because they increase the levels of insulin plus other types of food the most.

That's why it's always recommended eating healthy vegetable proteins and fats first, such as those provided by olive oil and avocado.

Protein gives you a longer feeling of satiety, as do vegetables and fats, which also reduces the production of ghrelin, and also gives you the necessary nutrients to maintain energy during the hours of fasting.

6º TOMAS EXCESS SNACKS

◆ ◆ ◆

You take excess snacks if you are one of those people who is allowed to take a mid-afternoon snack, or a small healthy snack in the middle of the window and food, we tell you that you are simply playing against it too.

You see, the digestive system takes a long time to process the food, absorb the nutrients and dispose of what it doesn't need.

During this time it not only burns calories but also keeps you satiated so your ghrelin levels do not increase and you do not suffer from hunger attacks as there is no stimulus to tell the body that it must eat.

But if you frequent to eat small snacks, no matter how healthy diet or ketogenic they may be, they still provide calories and indicate to the body that there is food to be consumed, so the ghrelin will make its appearance again to make you want more and more even though you don't really need it.

This is why many people feel an uncontrollable hunger in the middle of the afternoon, it is not because your body requires food, it is because the ghrelin is activated at that time thanks to the conditioning received and forces you to eat

This will logically also make the fasting hours and ghrelin active and make it more difficult to overcome the fasting, the best thing then is simply not to take a snack and wait until your dinner time to make a varied and satisfying full meal.

7º YOU TAKE COLLAGEN IN YOUR COFFEE KETO

◆ ◆ ◆

Keto coffee or bulletproof coffee, is a coffee that has become very popular among those who follow the ketogenic diet, has even crossed the borders Keto and is common to see it in the intermittent fasting.

This coffee is a mixture of black coffee with coconut oil or butter, to provide thanks to the body, many people break it helped in this way.

Some add peptides or hydrolyzed collagen supplements, to help the body maintain the production of collagen which improves the skin and muscle tissues and delays the onset of wrinkles.

Keto coffee with collagen is popular then but what you don't know, is that these collagen peptides are also amino acids that without carbohydrates can be transformed into sugar through a process known as gluconeogenesis, a way for the body to convert protein into glucose to obtain easy energy.

The problem with this is that collagen when converted into glucose, also raises the response to insulin, which ends up triggering other hormones such as ghrelin, and there in the hunger will become inclement.

Better try taking a collagen supplement in a shake that brings more nutrients to the body, or in water along with your heavy meal, but not in coffee.
That way you avoid the body taking it as glucose immediately.

8º YOU ARE NOT FLEXIBLE WITH YOUR FEEDING WINDOW

◆ ◆ ◆

Intermittent fasting can be inflexible, which means that it does not have to prevent you from sharing a meal with your friends.

A little food at a party or having to turn down a romantic evening just for fasting will not only make it hard for you to keep it up, but it will also take you away from your social circle.

To avoid this, you can play at making your fasting a little more flexible on special dates. To do this, all you have to do is calculate the times when you know you are going to eat for that different evening and square your eating window so that it is open during these hours.

For example, if you have a family dinner at 8pm but you know that everyone will end up eating at 9pm, then open your feeding window at 1pm instead of 12pm so you can share with your family, try this delicious recipe from your mom without having to sacrifice too much.

But of course, try to remember not to overdo it. Eat

your protein and vegetables first, and if you know there's a dessert coming up that you don't want to miss, try to make sure that the meals you eat during the day doesn't contain high levels of glucose.

It is always advisable to make your fasting a little more flexible, especially on special occasions, otherwise you will end up abandoning it and returning to your old consumption habits, which will make you gain weight again.

9º YOU DRINK ALCOHOL OUTSIDE YOUR FOOD WINDOW

◆ ◆ ◆

One mistake that almost all of us fall into at some point is giving ourselves permission to drink alcohol on an intermittent fast.

Whether in the fasting window, or in the eating window, we usually think of Cain alcoholic beverages as a kind of Bermuda triangle in the body, and that it does not affect weight or health.

But in reality all alcoholic drinks have calories, beer for example is a high calorie, high carbohydrate drink.

These are called empty calories because they make you gain weight, and they do not provide any kind of nutrient or benefit from a nutritional point of view.

Consuming alcohol during the feeding window, makes the organism concentrate on processing what is toxic to it to discard it, so it does not absorb the food or its nutrients well.

In addition, alcoholic beverages are an injection of pure glucose into the body that returns energy easily lost.

That's what prevents the fat-burning mechanism from being activated, and the worst thing is that the unburned calories from alcohol are then converted into more fat around the waist.

As the body was already warned that easy glucose can be available quickly ghrelin reappear during the fasting hours, or even stronger in the feeding window to ask you for more and more food.
That will make you desperately hungry, do you really want to lose all your effort just for a can of beer?

On the other hand, drinking alcohol during the fasting window directly breaks the fast, as it brings calories and carbohydrates into the body. This unbalances the whole fasting process in the body and you will have to start writing it up again.

It seems that it is already clear that alcohol in the intermittent fasting should not be an option.

10º YOU DON'T SLEEP ENOUGH

◆ ◆ ◆

The human organism needs rest to replenish its energy and repair any damage it may suffer during the day.

The problem is that most people have a penniless sleep level with only five or six hours of rest and often with insomnia and sleep interruptions.

When the body does not get enough rest, it cannot replenish its energy level to face the new day.

This causes the level of cortisol to rise, that famous stress hormone that makes us accumulate fat in the abdominal area every time we feel under attack which is almost all the time, due to the hectic lifestyle we lead.

The cortisol makes that also the ghrelin is seen, as the organism has not rested well, it does not obtain another form to obtain immediate energy and it looks for to take one of the foods quickly, by them it increases the sensation of hunger.

As a strategy to make you go for a slice of bread, the increase in cortisol and ghrelin together, I can make it very difficult to resist the hours of fasting, causing you to be in a bad mood and that the areas up to your window of feeding seem eternal.

To avoid this it is necessary to offer the body a rest time agreed, sleep between 7 and 8 hours per day is recommended, but you should also try to make it a continuous sleep relaxed and in a quiet environment so that anxiety or fear of strange noises cannot disturb you.

Practicing intermittent fasting is a healthy option to lose weight quickly. Review each of the errors that we have presented to you to determine which of them is negatively affecting your intermittent fasting.

Apply the necessary corrections, and you will soon feel better again, lose weight, and live a fuller, more productive life.

What do you think about these steps leave your comment,

Thank you for your review.

Jennifer J Collins

9 798671 179705